I0435252

Hello
My
Name
Is
Patricia
And
I
Am
An
Addict

A Handbook for Women and Men Battling Obesity and Morbid Obesity

By Patricia Ellis

Lulu Press Publishing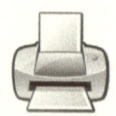

2019 by Patricia Ellis ISBN 978-0-359-33815-3

No part of this publication may be reproduced or transmitted in any form or by any

means without permission of the publisher. Unless otherwise indicated

© 2019 All rights reserved.

Cover Photo © Patricia Ellis Photography

Published by Lulu Press Publishing.

510-253-9108 Printed in the United States of America

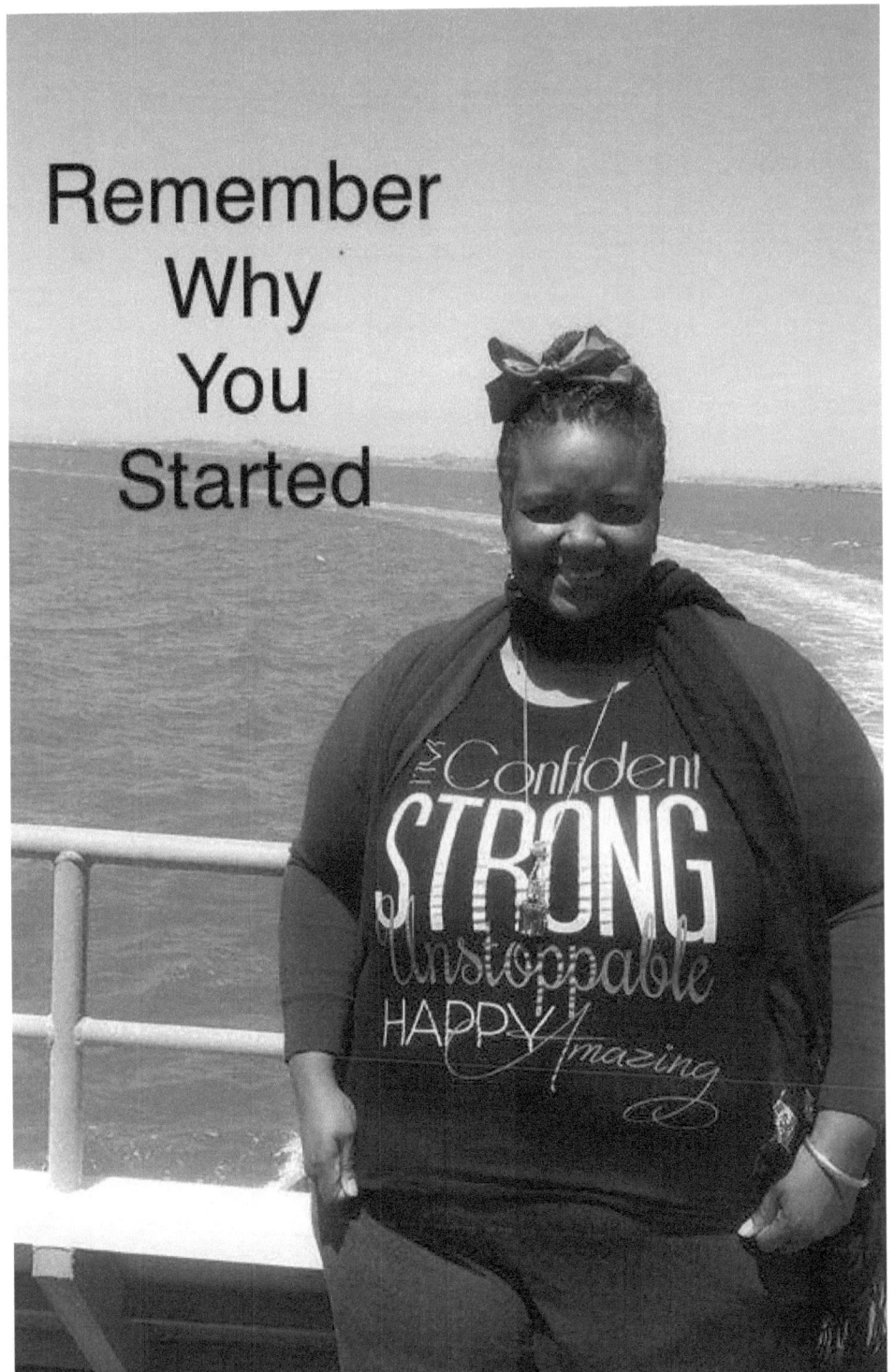

Remember
Why
You
Started

This book is for the 160 million people worldwide living with obesity or an unhealthy Body Mass Index Number. For the past 20 years I have been obese and tried over 100 diet plans, fads, green drinks, apple cider vinegars and fastings. And with no long term results. I have read so many books and attended boot camps. I still had no long term results. My heart attack I suffered inspired me to take action and seek answers on how I could be successful in breaking my addiction to sugar. I have successfully broke my addiction to sugar. This handbook is a A 30 Day Plan on How to Break the Addiction to Sugar and Live a Healthy Full Life. Being Active, Meditating, Praying, Reading your Bible and Living a Blessed Life.

PREFACE

During my twenty year addiction to sugar I masked 200 pounds of excess weight. I have talked with many people living with diseases and illnesses that are all weight related. Diseases such as heart disease, diabetes, high blood pressure, strokes, depression, heart attacks, thyroidism, cancer, eczema, hair loss, fibroids, PCOS, infertility, brain tumors and many other illnesses related to being overweight. I have always believed that being overweight was linked to a traumatic experience during your childhood. If you are someone you know has experienced a traumatic experience during your childhood and have not received therapy and have not healed from the truma, reach out to a medical professional right away. Get some help to get to a place of peace.

"Hello My Name Is Patricia And I am An Addict", is the product of my healing from bad decisions in my personal unhealthy habits of eating and inactivity. The simple thought of change in your daily routine causes anxiety. This 30 day pyramid plan handbook is designed to share all my potential pitfalls I faced in my battle to fight addiction. I am not a medical professional. Therefore always seek permission from your medical health care professional before you make any changes to your routine or nutritional intake.

Finally, this 30 day handbook is not a one size fits all book. This handbook focuses on methods you can use to break the addiction to sugar. Reading this handbook is the first step in taking action in breaking the chains of addiction.

The 30 Day Handbook Plan How to's Goals are to:

- *prevent medical and health problems related to obesity*
- *improve your understanding of addiction and obesity*
- *improve your ability to control your Body Mass Index.*

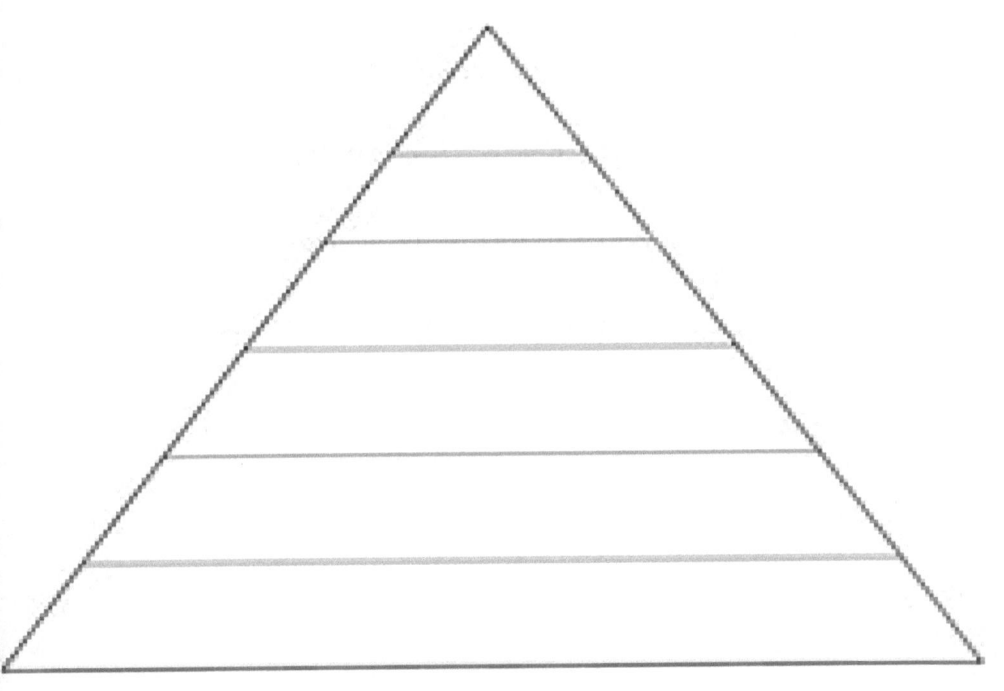

Patricia's 30 Day Food Pyramid Plan

To sum up weight gain and being overweight in two words: self control. Diet plans make some true and some unrealistic expected results. I will share my own personal pitfalls and a 30 day plan to break the addiction cycle to sugar. Where do I begin? In 2018 or 1998? Well for time sake I will start in 1998 when my overeating began and the why behind my over eating. When if you read my last book " Now That I Know , Now What" you know that I have a bad habit of ignoring the warning signs to unhealthy relationships which includes food.

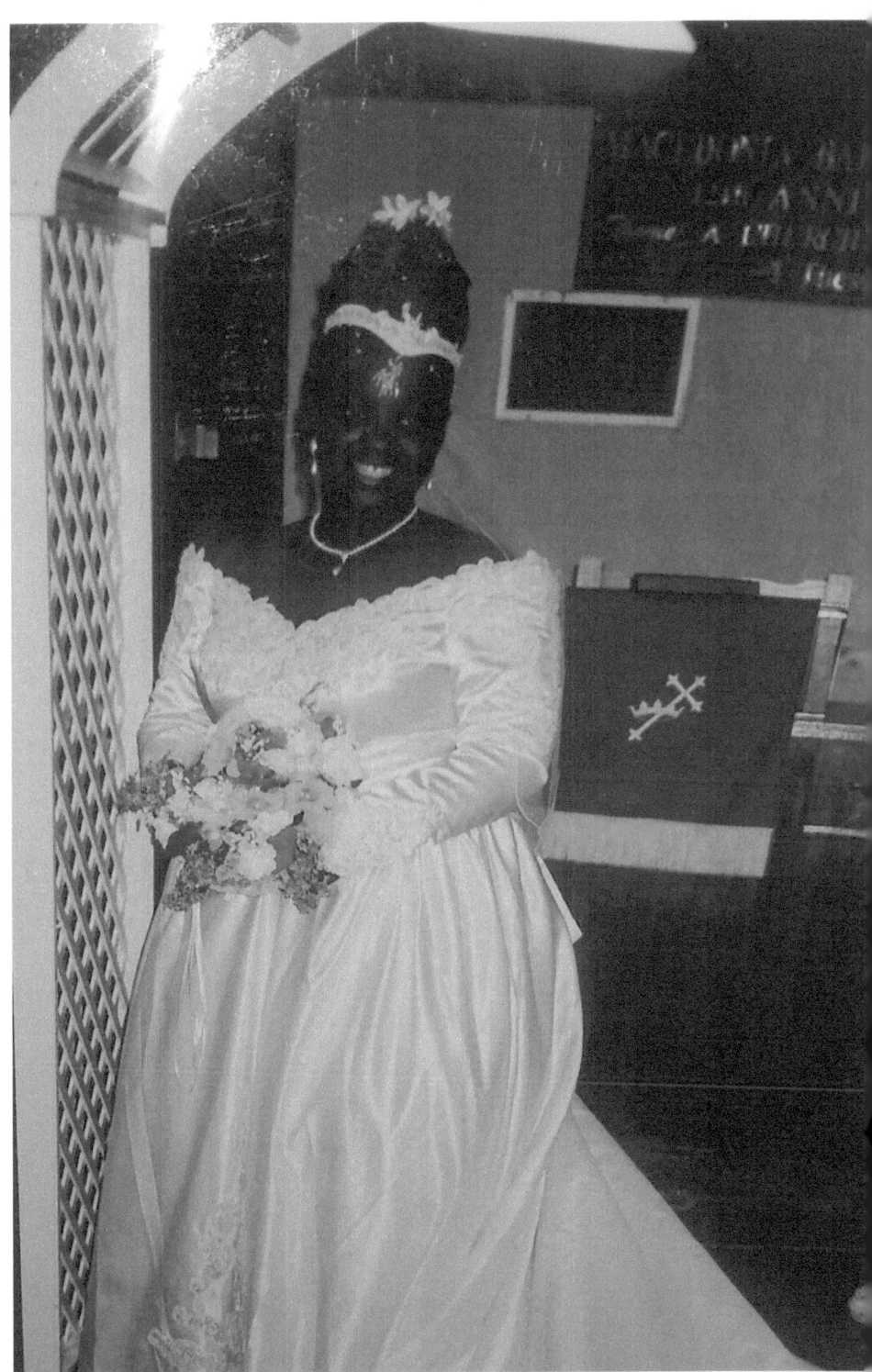

Eugene Jones

From our Monday through Friday routine of spending
money on eating at fine dining restaurants and take out
eateries is when the upward number on the scale began.
In 1998 I had the perfect figure. A slim waist, tight
thighs. perfectly shaped hips, muscular arms, perfect abs
and no belly fat. I was a stay at home wife to the perfect
husband. Until, reality sat in. Yep reality. I would shop at
at Hilltop Mall, travel to any destination I desired and I
had it all. So I thought. I was so busy taking care and
making sure my husband had his clothes ironed, hair cut,
lunch prepared, new cars and all his hearts desires. I
forgot to care about myself. I did not have a gym

membership or a personal trainer. I omitted my needs and my desires. I noticed my hips started to spread at first. So, I started to walk up and down Hilltop Mall Road and walk the entire Rolling Hills Cemetery. Our homeowners association had a pool so I would go there when it was warm to play and walk in the water.

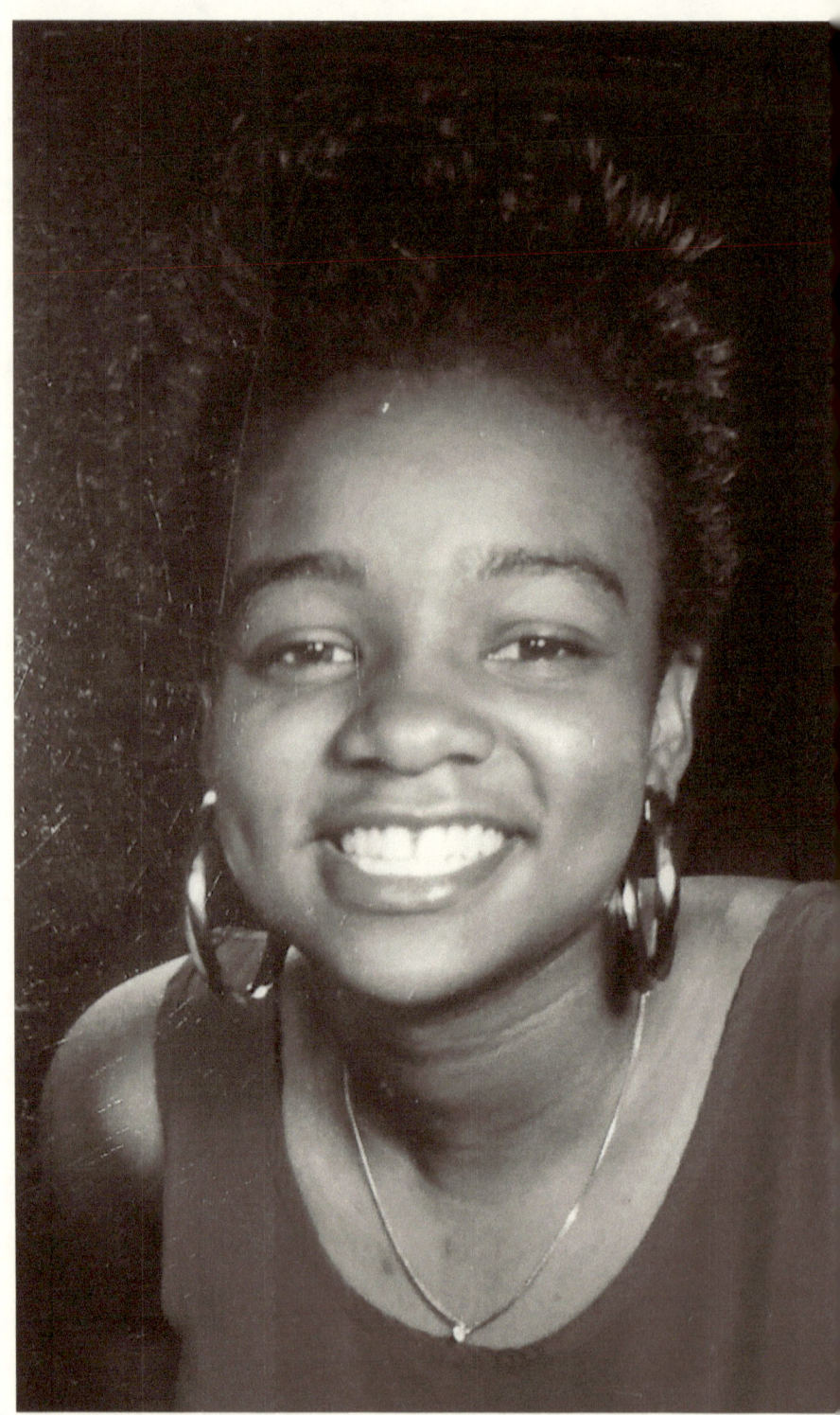

What led to further weight gain? A cheating and lying husband! Yes but thats my next book. Have you ever been perfect for your husband or your wife? You do any and every thing in your power to be the so called trophy wife. I dressed in tight dresses and shorts. I wore halter tops and high heels. Yup, I was only 20 and had a new husband. So you know it went down. We both were young, vibrant and excited about all the new things we will experience together. Eating was on the top on my list for my husband. He loved fried pork chops, jiffy cornbread and green beans. This was his favorite dinner meal in which he ate at 8:00 am the time he got off work from the United States Postal Service. I know you wanna hear the juicy part right? Well here it goes. A family member got my husband hooked on drugs. Who? Which family member? Well I will leave that for another book too. But, I will say that people are jealous and they will devour who and what you love simply because you have and they do not. It's that simple. When Eugene and I were finally divorced and going on dates again he said he could never get back in a relationship with me because my family was like poison. I told him that he was warned about some of the people in my family. Many of my family members were career criminals and I advised and pleaded with him to stay away from them. Eugene made the choice to entertain and indulge in their demise of his own self destruction. Wait, I am calling the kettle black and I was living right in the house with him self destructing like a time bomb. I was not taking care of my health and my weight skyrocketed. We ate more and we ate more. We had lavish parties, road trips all over the US. We had so many family events I lost count. Our home was the house where everyone came to have a good time. Everyone except me. I had the American

Dream: Homeowner, Married, New Cars, Money in the bank, American Express card with no limit. When I say I was living the no limits life. Until Eugene went out cheating. One chick egged our new 1999 White Ford Ranger truck, keyed f you b all over my new 2000 Ford Explorer and the same chick left her diabetes needles in our 2000 Ford Mustang. Damn, did I think I would get married, buy a home and live happily ever after hell naw. How could I focus on me and my health if I got all this going on in my life and I am only 20. How did I get here? Get where? Get to 180lbs. Drama, Lies and lack of Self Control. I can not continue in the vicious cycle of blaming others for my lack of self control. I am 20 and can not control what I put in my mouth. I could have what I wanted to eat and when ever I wanted to eat. I was a pig. I mean I really was a pig in gluteney. I ate food high in sodium and high in sugar. I had no regards for myself. How did I get here? I did not take the time for myself. Many women of all ages cater and meet the needs of everyone and everything else other than themselves. Did you take 10 minutes for yourself today with no distractions ? Free from your spouse, kids and your family members. A few months had passed and I began to work for a local mortgage company. And if you know anything about real estate you know that mortgage and real estate organizations eat out a lot for business meeting and mixers. They also go on lavish vacation and snow trips. By Lavish I mean highly saturated fats, meats, dairy and sweets. Everyday I indulged in donuts, chocolate, cookies, cakes, pies. What we cooked at work in crockpots were beef stews. They were so good I can still remember the savory of the salt from the beef. This unhealthy relationship and lack of self control lasted all the way until 2018. I would get on and off sugar. I would get right and follow a well balanced 1350 calories and drink my 1 gallon of water. Until I was triggered and I would relapse. Maybe I was the only one with a favorite oversized spoon and a huge bowl the size of a large cantaloupe and it was red in color for my cereal. When you lack self control you pick up everyone else's bad habits. As a child and an adult I never ate Captain Crunch cereal. But when your husband loves that cereal you eat it even if you do not like it.

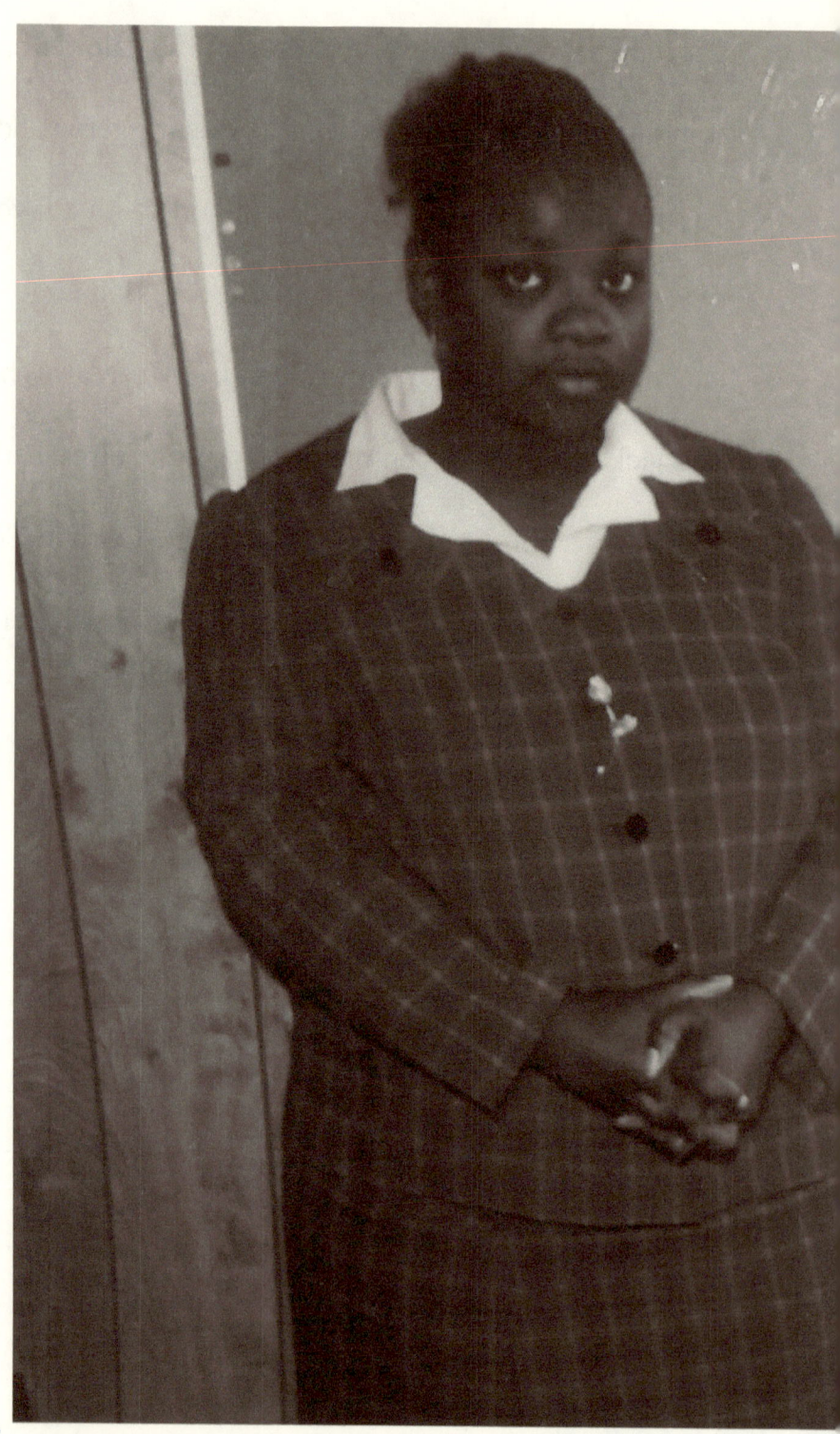

Honestly, lack of self control is hazardous. Binge eating and eating based on emotions will have you weighing 0.15 of a ton over time. This seems like the same story over and over again. It is and it's an addiction. Millions of people all over the globe are addicted to something. It may not be drugs, alcohol, sex, money or even food. But most are addicted to something. What's an addict? Someone that lacks self control or self discipline to not commit an act or task. Now I know why addiction is so hard to break. It's because of your self discipline has to be structured and support system must be very strong and enforceable in a way. How did I break the addiction? Well, honestly I have failed hundreds of times over the past 20 years. I tried and joined Jenny Craig and Weight

Watchers. I have tried the atkins diet, military diet, cabbage diet, green smoothie diet, water only diet, no meat diet, liquids only diet, bootcamps and personal trainers. I have joined 24 hour Fitness, Bally Fitness, East Oakland Sports Center and the YMCA. I have tried meal planning and I have even had a personal chef come to my home multiple time to try and jump start my dead self-care cell in my life battery.

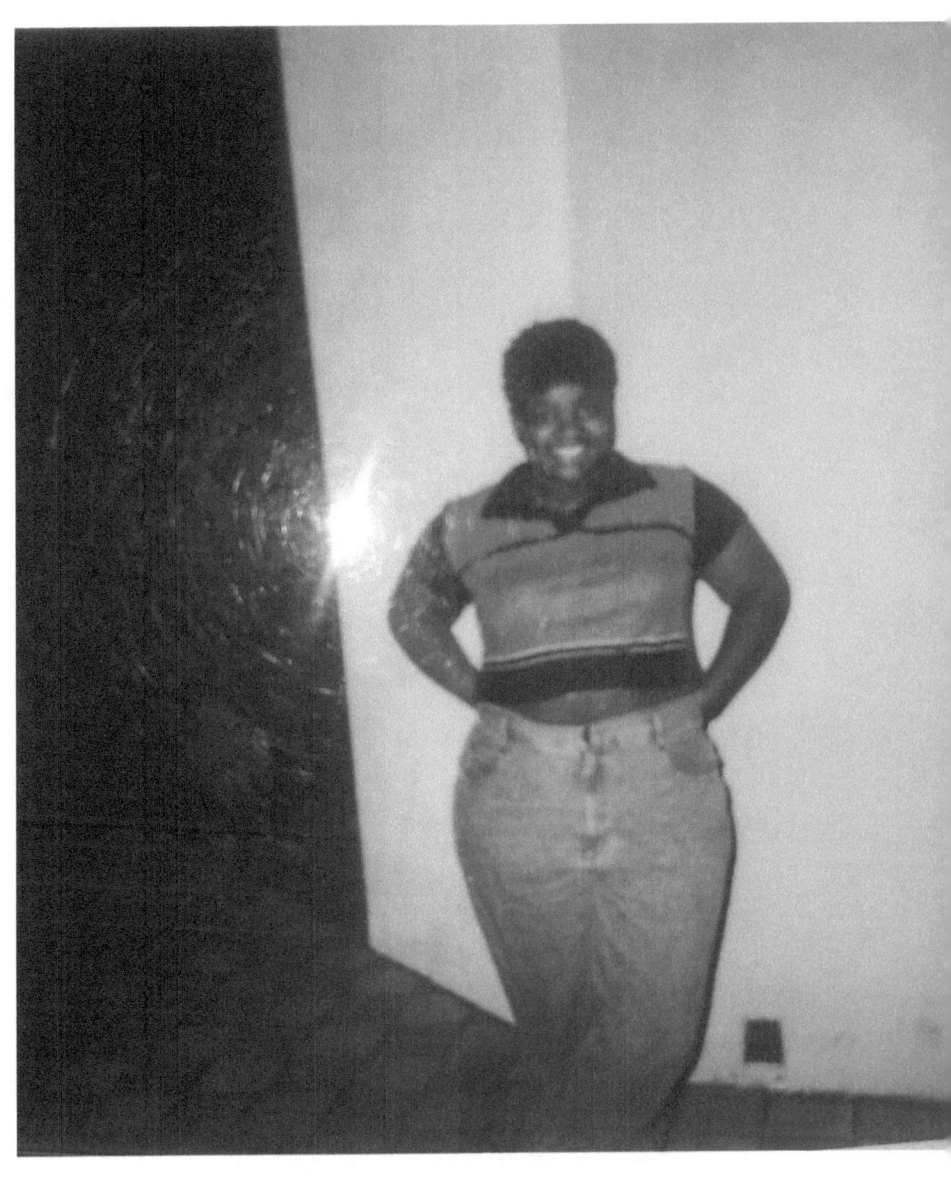

Being overweight is no joke and the pitfalls I faced on

the addiction of 20 years were very common. However,

with pain comes addiction. It took me over 20 years to come to the conclusion that addiction is linked to pain. 200lbs of pain to be exact is what I carried around as my addiction. I had self inflicted addiction cause by all the hurt, pain, setbacks and brokenness I faced. Pitfall is when you have the opportunity to make the right choice. However based on unhealed emotions you walk right up to the dark and dry pit and you jump in. Pits are dangerous and hazardous to your life expectancy results. If you live in or have ever visited the San Francisco Bay Area you have witnessed what addiction looks like. As a teen we often visited the local corner store for chips and candy. Each time I would visit this corner store a man about the age of 40, would stand in front of the corner store drinking his Old English 800 beer. This man would yell and stream derogatory words to all that entered the store. As I got older I continued to visit the store. About

15 years had passed and this man was still drinking his

beer in front of the corner store. Except this time he was

in a wheelchair and one of his legs had been amputated.

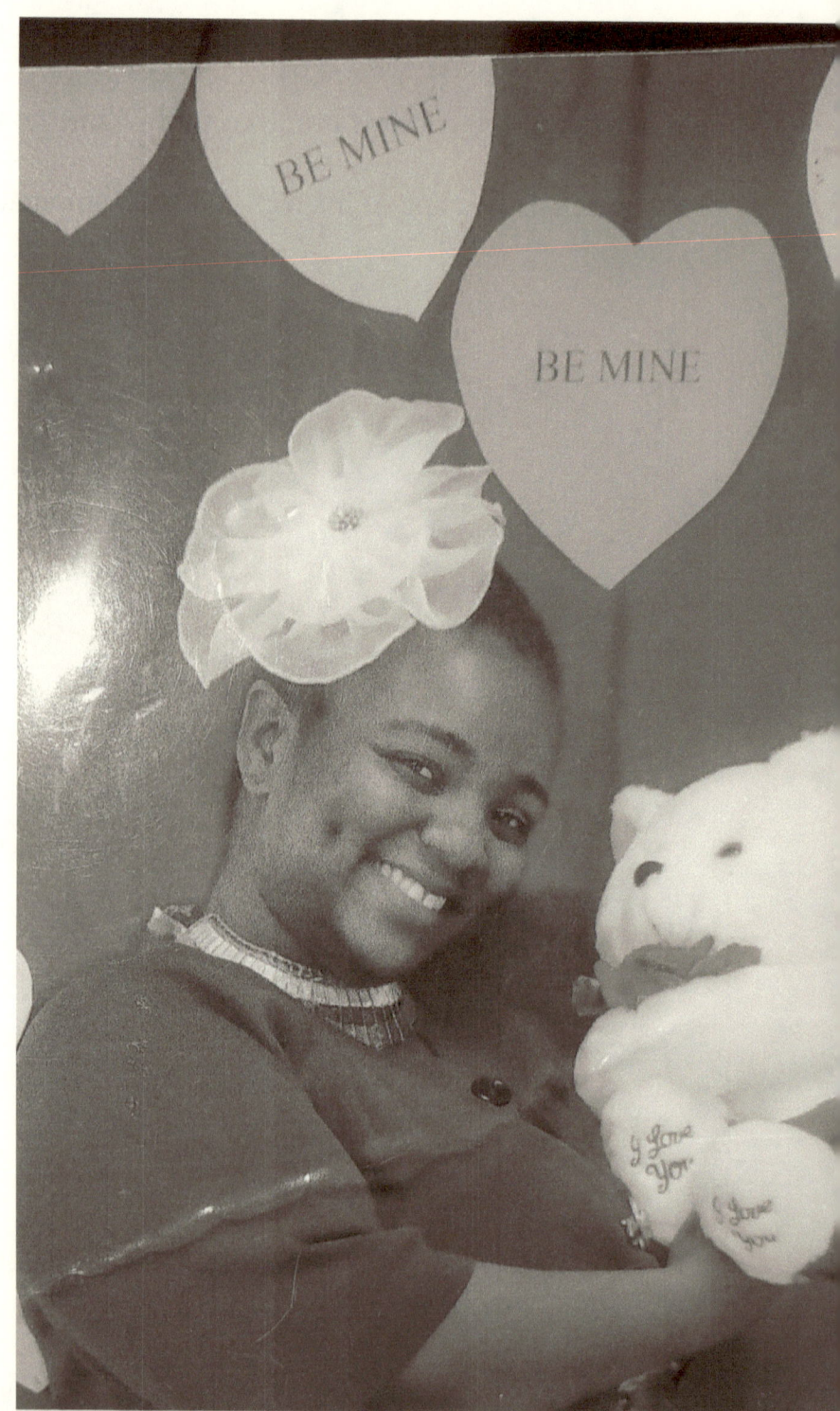

Earlier I had talked about illnesses linked to obesity.

Well addictive behavior leads to obesity.

This 30 day plan is not going to solve all the unresolved issues you may have if you are obese. Stop wasting your health plan coverage use it. Call and talk to a therapist, dietitian, nutritionist, psychiatrist, psychologist, social worker, wellness coach, doctor or many other highly skilled and equipped to give you all the tools to break the addiction. I did.

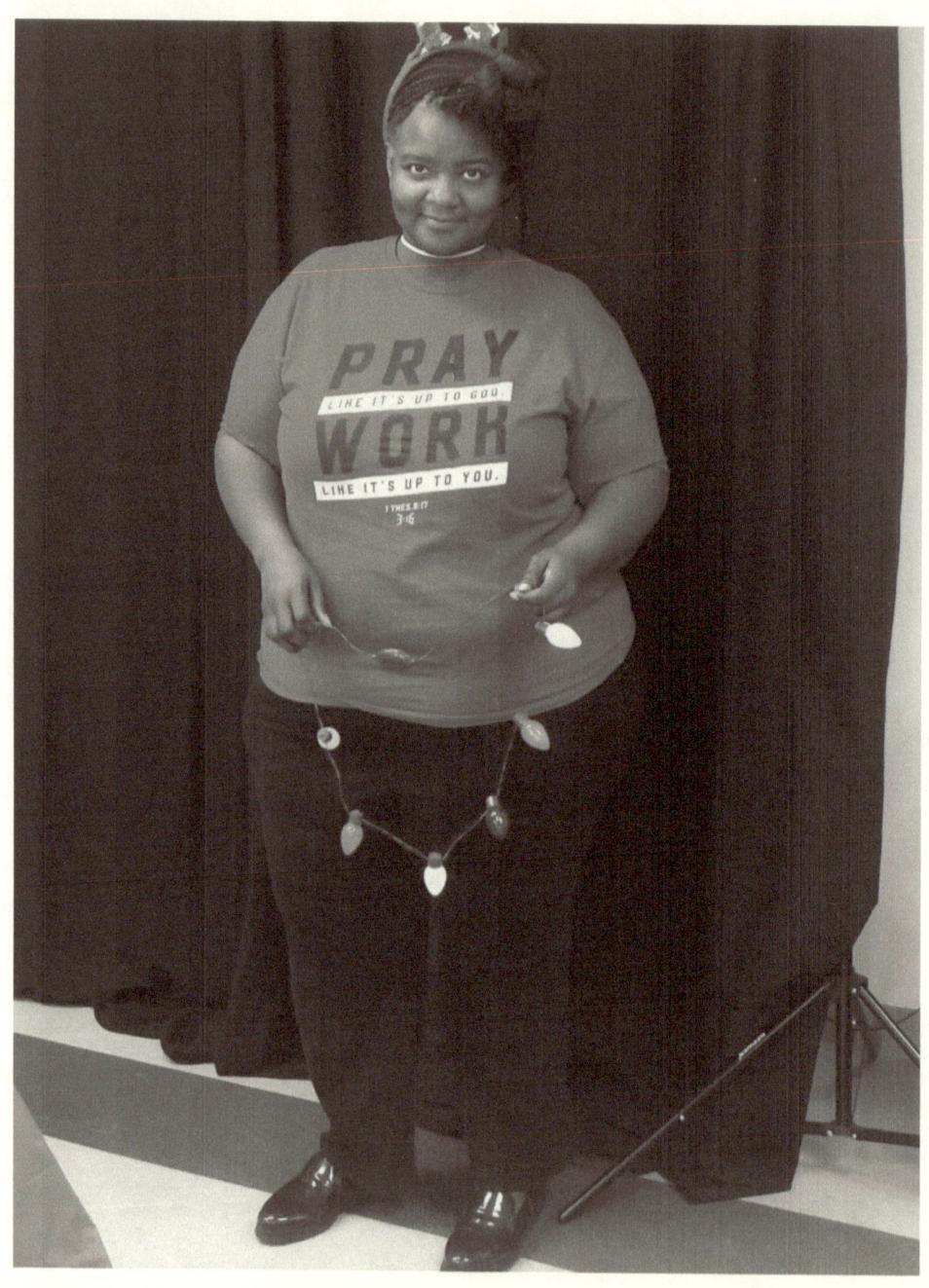

There is so much power in the daily affirmations in I AM. Everyday you have to start off with at least 10 - I AM Positive Affirmations. I AM……….

I AM NOT ADDICTED TO FOOD

I WILL MEET ALL MY GOALS TODAY

I WILL MAKE HEALTHY CHOICES

I WILL EXERCISE

I WILL EAT TO LIVE

I WILL CONTROL WHAT I PUT IN MY MOUTH

I AM A BRICK HOUSE

I AM A STRONG WOMAN/MAN

I WILL BREAK THE ADDICTION TO unhealthy FOOD

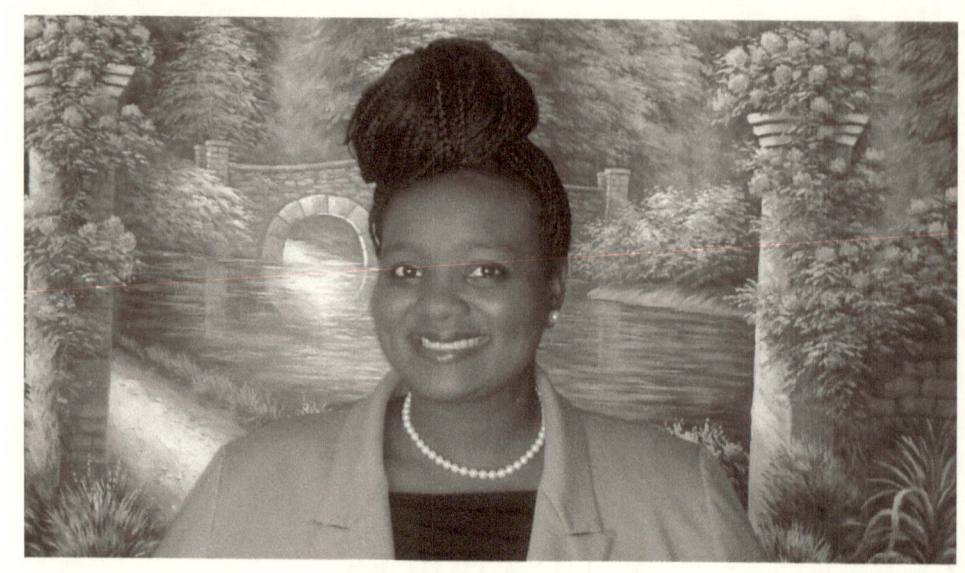

FRIENDSHIPS

Friendships are also vital to breaking the addiction to unhealthy eating. Over the past 20 years I have had some friends. Friends that build up and some friendame's that tear down. Friends that I have prayed with for hours. Friendame's that have said all manner of evil against me. I have one friend name Chantia we have been Sisters in Christ for over 35 years. We still meet on our monthly girls meet up at the top eateries to talk about God's goodness and his mercy towards us. Some of my childhood friends have gone their on way and we message each other on social media. My friend since 1996 Sister Swameka we still meet occasionally and share God's realness in our lives. We support each other in ministry. Friends how many of us have them? Do you have a friend that you can depend on? A friend that will cover you and check you too? Do you have a friend that will walk the marina with you? Do you have a friend that will tell you straight up ? I have a friend and the told me straight up with no chaser. "Tricia I know you have had some things happen to you over your life and you need to get some help so you can get back to being a healthier you" ! My response was silence at first. I knew my BMI was off the chart literally. Then I responded with tears. I cried and I cried. We hugged and the rest is history. I got it! It took someone else to acknowledge, face me and tell me what they saw. Wait what! Put the book down and go grab a mirror or go stand in the bathroom mirror. What did you see? A smiling face. Or did you see sagging arms, saddle bag hips, 3 row stomach, love handles, chunky cheeks? Now go get the scale. Go and weight yourself. What did the scale read? Are you in your normal BMI? Mostly likely if you are reading this book you are overweight and you can not get your weight under control.

You are not alone. The next few pages will guide you with 5 STEPS on how to get back to that normal healthy Body Mass Index.

<u>Try this plan for 30 days</u>......

Email me when you reach your health goals

<u>EllisForOakland@gmail.com</u>

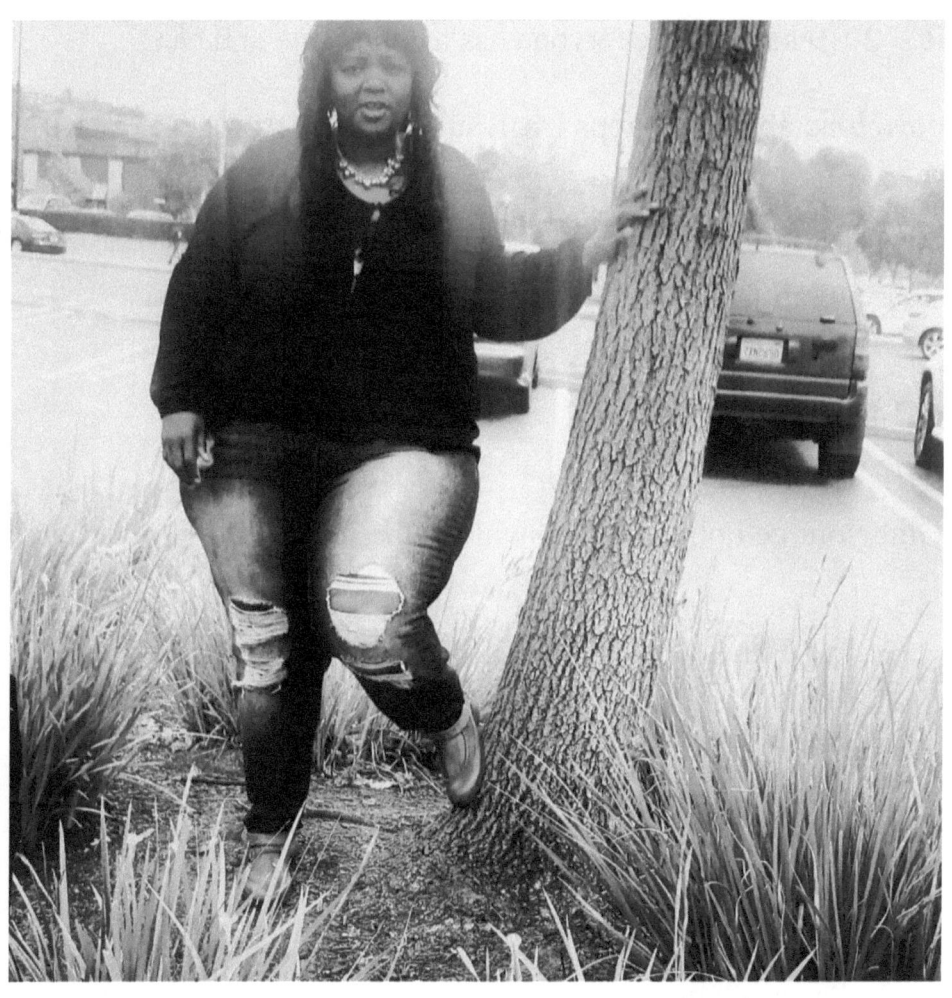

It's 2019 so almost everyone has a cell phone and can download apps. The apps I will suggest worked for me. There are hundreds of apps you can try. But, at least try these because these are all free:

STEP 1

Grab your cell phone and download the four apps below

1. My Fitness Pal- Track your calories to eat a balanced and healthy meal -Also free blog post to motivate you daily. You can also join walking and fitness challenges weekly to challenge yourself.

2. Pacer- Counts your steps to reach your 10,000 steps daily goal. You can set up hourly reminders to get moving when inactive.

3. Aqua Alert- Counts your daily water intake and set up hourly reminders to reach your water intake daily goals.

4. Google Calendar- Calendar to schedule all your fitness and exercise activities

STEP 2

Meet with your medical doctor in person

1. Bring a list of all your health concerns

Be real honest with yourself and leave nothing out. For example

Left shoulder pain-left ankle pain when walking- irregular bowel movements-unstable emotions-unprotected sex with multiple partners-drug use with shared needles- weight gain over 50lbs-100lbs-200lb-300lbs-400lbs-500lbs-600lbs- sexual assault- sexual abuse- domestic violence- mental health

STEP 3

Set realistic health goals- example make healthy choices when faced with triggers daily- Trigger examples may include: Kids acting up, spouse not coming come, overworked, dog barking, traffic on the freeway, financial hardship, family drama, family scandals, family embarrassment, food not pre-made, fast food is more convenient, you breakup with your mate, your parent dies, your child dies, you lose your job, you become homeless, you relocate and many more other trigger.

Realistic goals include but not limited to:

Drink a ½ of a bottle of water every 30 minutes

Walk - even if it's in place every 20 minutes

Attend your therapy appointments weekly to aid in your healing the pain from the addiction to food

STEP 4 Journaling

Journal- At the end of every single day -sit down and write out all your feelings from the current day. Journaling will help to identify triggers in your life that have led to addictive eating behavior. Find you a cute journal at a Michael's craft store they have over 20 to choose from and they are only $5 each.

5. PLAN a MONTHLY FOOD and ACTIVITIES CALENDAR

Example Meal Plan

Breakfast:

 2 Veggies- 1 protein

Scrambled Eggs -2 max or 2 boiled eggs

 1 piece of Fish/Chicken baked

Lunch:

2 Veggies -1 Seafood or Chicken or Fish

1 cup of cooked Spinach

1 Small baked Yam

1 piece of baked Salmon

Dinner

Baked or Grilled Chicken Caesar Salad

A small bowl of green bean or black eye peas

1 piece of whole grain wheat bread- toasted

Snacks:

Fresh fruit 2 max per day of your choice

1 avocado and 1 spoonful of peanut butter

Apple/Banana/Kiwi/Blueberries/Orange/Pear

Drinks: Water- A Minimum of 1 gallon per day

30 DAY EXERCISE PLAN to met your 10,000 steps each day

SUNDAY- Walk at your local lake, marina or park for a

minimum of 90 minutes

MONDAY- Walk your local mall for 45 minutes

TUESDAY- Exercise with a youtube video fitness for 45 minutes

WEDNESDAY-Walk your local beach

THURSDAY-Attend a community exercise class

FRIDAY-Attend a community meditation class

SATURDAY-Hike at your local hiking trail

Are you looking for the rest of the plan? Put the book down again a grab a mirror! What did you see in the mirror? You!

You are fitting piece to the puzzle. You hold the key to unlock and free your peace and happiness. I need you do something else for you. Find a random key you no longer use and place it on your choice of a lancet and wear the key around your neck starting right now. Wear it like its your id badge for work.

Without this key you can not gain access to unlock what's holding you bondage in addictive behavior which has led to your obesity. You hold the key to true happiness in your own life. You have to make the decision to not be a puppet like elmo being controlled by triggers. Read this aloud. I WILL NOT BE A PUPPET ANYMORE. I WILL CONTROL WHAT GOES IN MY MOUTH EVERYTIME MY MOUTH OPENS. I CHOSE TO BE HAPPY. I WILL NO LONGER ALLOW MY BAD DECISIONS AND CHOICES TO STEAL MY CONTROL. I CAN AND I WILL LOSE THIS WEIGHT. I WILL SURROUND MYSELF WITH ACTIVE PEOPLE. I WILL VISIT MY DOCTOR REGULARLY. I AM A WINNER. I WILL MEET ALL MY GOALS I SET OUT TO REACH. I WILL BE POSITIVE ON PURPOSE. I CONTROL EVERY FOOD ON MY PERSONAL FOOD PYRAMID. I WILL START MY 30 DAY PLAN TO BREAK MY ADDICTION TO FOOD.

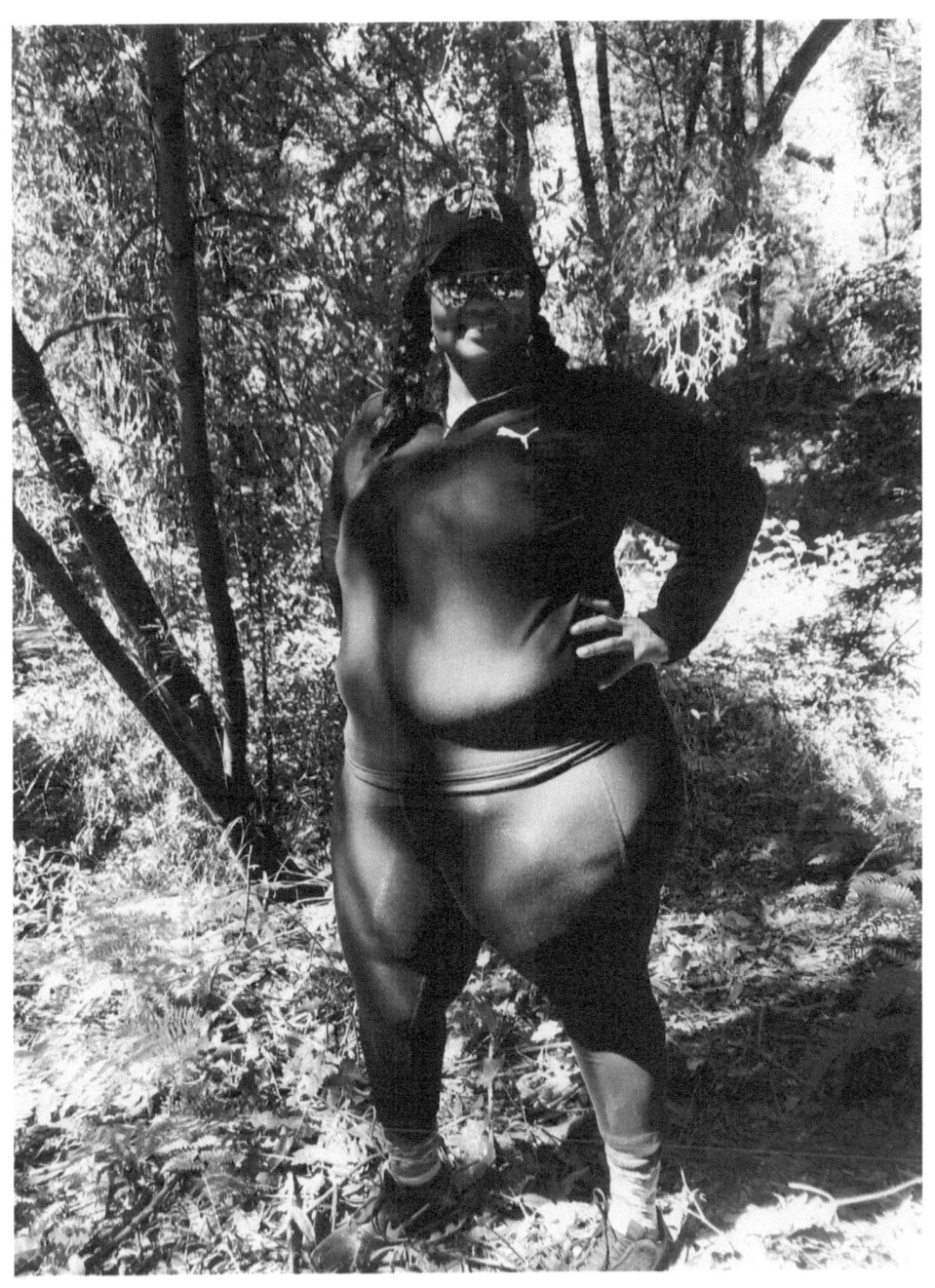

Just a reminder…. here are a few health illnesses that are linked to being overweight and obese.

Stroke   *Heart Attack*   *Brain Tumor*

High Blood Pressure   Infertility PCOS   Arthritis   Limited Mobility

Kidney Failure   Depression   Diabetes

Now that you have all the information on how to set goals and reach them. What will you do to take action in your own life?

I pray that I continue the 30 Day Plan to live a long life healthy.

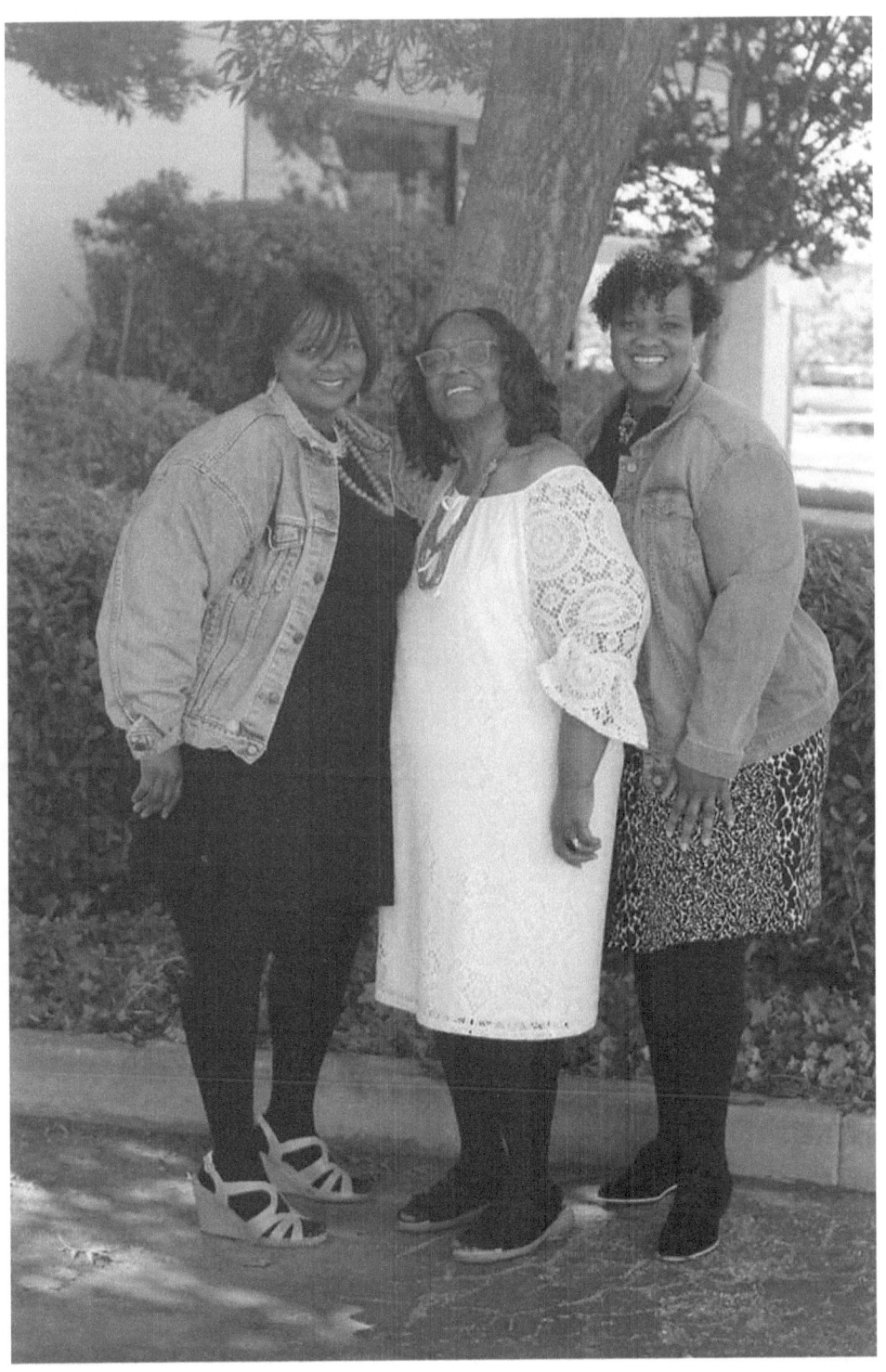

RESOURCES FOR THE 160 Million Worldwide Battling Obesity

OverEaters Anonymous www.oa.org

Offers in person and virtual online resources and support for overeating and undereating, food addiction, bulimia, binge eating and over exercising.

SUPPORT GROUPS For Those Obese

https://obesity.supportgroups.com/

Over 42,000 members in the online support group

Alameda County Public Health Alameda County Diabetes Program

The Diabetes Program provides self-management classes to adults diagnosed with pre-diabetes and Type 2 diabetes.

www.ingramcontent.com/pod-product-compliance
Lightning Source LLC
Chambersburg PA
CBHW031334290526
45784CB00014B/2714